To KENNI SPENCER

To know you was to love you,
To love you was to honor you,
To honor you was a privilege,
Always friends,
For ever sweet hearts.

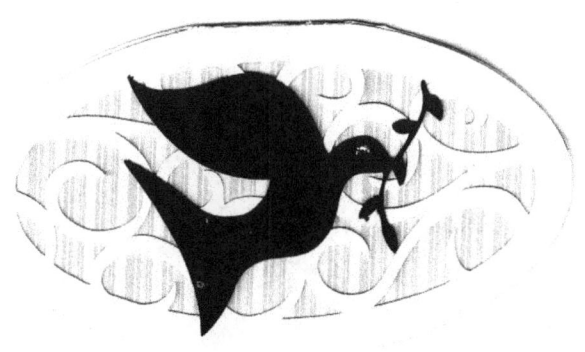

CONTENTS

I WATCH AND I CRY: A BRAIN IN A CHAIR
Living, loving, and caring for a soul mate with ALS

We had just gotten back from an exciting adventure in the Eagle Cap wilderness in late June of 2008. Our lives were changing in that retirement was ebbing into our thoughts and so there was much discussion.

Life just seems to crank on and no one thinks about a life changing event. We tend to think about living life and wait for the next process to grip our mind and reactions. Most of us never prepare for anything except living in and through our family and friends sphere of influence.

Shortly after returning from our Eagle Cap trip, my wife Kenni, started to complain about buttoning her shirt and how it was becoming difficult moving her right hand. Life just went on, as it does at our age when you put-up with the nuances of getting older suffering with pains and aches. Her condition continued to get worse, after which we decided to make a doctor visit.

Little did we know this life changing event was upon us encircling our whole being. The beginning of many doctor visits and finally a diagnosis of carpal tunnel/ulnar nerve damage from a horse fall on our Eagle Cap trip...successful surgery and finally relief. Oh how sweet it is!

The relief was short lived, in that through rehabilitation, the condition was not improving but rather continuing to degrade. There were more and more things that Kenni could not do with her right hand and arm. More doctor visits and more tests while continuing to have more troubles with her right hand and arm.

MRI's, nerve conductions tests, blood tests, brain scans. Wow unbelievable! Some showed that there were nerve conduction problems but a good brain MRI. After the final general practioner consult, Kenni came home elated that the brain MRI was clean and her relieved response to me; "You're not going to get rid of me, I am here for the duration". That day we bathed in the good news and celebrated...it would now just take more time to heal than we anticipated. God is good!

Six months later after returning from visiting our youngest son in New Zealand, Kenni started noticing issues with her left hand and some slurring speech. Panic has now set in...we initiated more doctor visits at the best neurological clinics in the area. Never a diagnosis, but a scary consult...WE SUSPECT MOTOR NEURON CONDITION. Finally in April of 2009 a diagnosis of ALS (Lou Gehrig's disease)...what? Are you kidding me!

A vibrant being struck hard,
Selfless, loving, bound to a chair,
The biggest fight of her life is in store
What are we going to do?

Kenni and Family have now entered into this unknown journey. Unknown in that we have only heard of Lou Gehrig's disease, but never given it a second of thought. What is ALS and what can you take to make it go away or control it? There has got to be a pill! There has got to be a treatment! Kenni has contracted a rare, but increasing occurrence disease. Only 30,000 people are afflicted with ALS each year in the US. It is a fatal disease according to the American medical community. What…2-5 years of life? What kind of life? Oh, I better do some research about this thing to find out what she can take to make her better! Everything will be fine and she will get better, that's for sure.

This life story journey is purely from my perspective, Kenni's husband, companion, lover and soon to be committed caregiver. I need to get this written down for me and only me. It's about what I see, what I feel, what I experience, and what I do in responding to the conditions this disease manifests itself in. How this surprise evilness sneaks into everyone's life and makes you think, feel and act completely different than you ever thought or have done in the past. Incredible anger and unbelievable sadness takes over my soul. Explaining to you what I feel, see, experience, and do is what gives you the essence of living with a soul mate having ALS; truly A BRAIN IN A CHAIR, but yet a loving, caring, vibrant brain at that.

Your stuck can't change things,
Try to move but can't,
It's like wrapped in cellophane,
Weep all the time and multiple victims

Since Kenni's whole career life was spent as an educator, she would request that I offer an outline first before explaining this BRAIN IN A CHAIR JOURNEY to you:

I. HOW CAN WE AFFORD TO LIVE WITH THE EXPENSE OF TREATING THIS DISEASE

II. HOW WILL THIS DISEASE IMPACT HER LIFE PASSIONS OF TEACHING, QUILTING, AND FAMILY

III. WATCHING THE DISEASE LIVE AND EFFECT LIFE

IV. FAMILY LIVING WITH THE DISEASE

V. PROVIDING CARE WHILE TRYING TO LIVE A "NORMAL LIFE"

VI. FAMILY AND FRIENDS

VII. THE FINAL CHAPTER

Well that's about the essence of the BRAIN IN A CHAIR journey outline. I will do my best to stick to the outline. By the way, my only goal in writing this is to help me and give others insights into a real face of ALS! I hope that it can make me feel better. I hope that this effort can make my anger go away and soothe my soul somewhat. I hope that it gives insights to others the impact of the attack of ALS within a family.

Like some people, our retirement was to continue to work as long as we could physically, while continuing to help our children. People who know Kenni; her children were her first priority and her students second. All the rest of "family" was there to love and experience life. Our retirement planning, like many, was retirement income, our home, social security, a home quilting business and her husband's business. That should about do it...not a lot but we will get by. Out of nowhere a big evil disease has wrapped its tentacles around us sucking the life out of each and every one of us. It is truly spirit killing! Now begins the task of dealing with Social Security before 65, medical expense issues, and setting up doctor networks and just figuring out how to pay the daily bills. Wow, this is overwhelming trying to understand the rules of governmental bureaucracy and how they apply here.

When you get in a "crunch situation", trying to collect and understand all the necessary information is not only difficult, but very frustrating. You can't obtain all the information from one source or one phone call. This applies to not only to the labyrinth of medical information, but insurance and governmental stuff as well.

The person, who is sick, generally can't always be at the "top of their game" and offer the best help.

Dealing with Social Security is like dealing with a prosecuting attorney, who knows that you are guilty of cheating before even meeting and knowing you. Since too many people have abused this system of Social Security Disability, the process is frightful, stressful and frustrating. No wonder "pre-old people" are cranky! There are rules for everything and time lines for everything. Guess what, the rules and timelines do not mesh with yours - period! How about that! The Washington State Disability System was the most friendly to deal with. Why is that? The Federal Government is absolutely the worst...what a bureaucratic nightmare! You are still dealing with people, whose only function is to do their job, then go home at 5:00pm to their families. The check marks they make in the boxes, they have no clue the huge impact that it makes on your life.

Our goal was simple in this first phase of the journey...maintain our current standard of living and live our lives as NORMALLY as we could... (Eat well, laugh, love and pay the bills).

The second phase was to slow the progression of this evil disease and the final phase was to get something back that the disease had taken away. Clearly, this was a tall order. In these early stages, it is still very easy to not give up and continue to charge ahead.

This process took 8 months to finalize and take effect. After the April 2009 diagnosis, it was in February 2010 that we clearly understood our financial status. We were not prepared for this long time line financially. Kenni took her third retirement from Clark College in June 2009. Washington State Disability kicked in October of 2009. Kenni's Federal Social Security Disability kicked- in February 2010. Mike decided to take his Social Security in November 2009, early but you have to do what makes sense. Now, what's this medical insurance thing all about?

Since the money time lines were all different we elected to take Cobra through Clark College…wow that's expensive…triple what our original medical premiums were. Clearly, this was the best short term course to take. How can we afford this? Ya know, you just do and try to get by. But it really hurt us financially. Money tends to be the root of some evil. It begins to become as important as the disease. Anger seeps slowly into your psyche. Since we had absolutely done no planning for a terminal disease, the future was very uncertain.

Again, you are sort of behind the eight ball, and time is of the essence. If you don't meet the necessary insurance time-lines, then it can take months to be able to secure qualification. If this happens and you do not have adequate savings, this could bankrupt you, creating a financial disease.

Next is Medicare (hundreds of different plans); Providence, Medicare Advantage, AARP, Blue Cross, Kaiser…on and on. Then there is a Supplemental healthcare plan necessary, a drug plan…and I am sure more. There was research, research, research, and more research to select the best plan which is most affordable and fits your needs. Do you pick one that has low co-pays, but higher deductibles or vice versa? What about hospital stays, drug coverage, eye, dental, alternative medicine? When can you change plans? Oh boy!!HELP!! By the way there is none that will fit into our time frame…it's only you who can and want to help. Everyone has their own situation and problems, so getting good advice is hard to get. With ALS, the State and Federal Governments have waived Medicare and Social Security with early acceptance. This was a very important thing thanks to the ALS Societies lobbying in Washington DC. At least something positive has surfaced. However, picking the right supplemental insurance plan for this disease was frightful. Again, ya do what ya have to do and pick the best you can…we did, Medicare as primary and Washington Uniform Medical as secondary. Wow, I hope that is right! Did I make the right decision? I don't know! Just run with it!

One of the biggest struggles during this phase was that Kenni's disease relegated her to minimal help. She could not sign documents, could not speak to be understood, and could not control her emotions well enough to respond and help make decisions. As we were dealing with the Federal Social Security regime over the phone, both of us had to be on the phone responding to questions...guess what, Kenni could not speak to be understood. Therefore, we had to physically meet with the Social Security regime, and they wanted to ask questions and sign documents...she could not do this! I have to admit that the Social Security experience is one of the "coldest" receptions ever. You take a number to "queue-up" for your meeting. The people were totally non-emotional regarding your situation. Oh well, now's the time for Power of Attorney! What the heck is all this about? Then Kenni cries...how does a stranger respond to this type of behavior? As you can see, more and more of this process were falling upon my shoulders. I might add that one of the greatest strengths of Kenni was dealing with the administrative minutia of our family life...taking care of the family details and running of the house hold. I cooked, worked, and mowed lawns. This is not my forte!! But...I have got to do this...very stressful I might add and all of this outside of my comfort-zone. This starts to reflect in increased anger, impatience, and aggressiveness...traits that make you truly seem cranky and old.

As we continued to live fighting, thanks to my parents…there was a little help in cash flow management on the medical insurance bill side. I got it paid back but it took a while. It is very hard to reach out for financial support when your 62 years old, assuming your parents are still alive. Kenni's mom really helped after she died, since Kenni was the executor of the estate. This inheritance really provided a needed cushion. One of the major emotions is that we have been so quietly independent and confident about our life direction, that reaching out for help at our age is extremely hard to do when it involves money. We are not kids, but rather "pre-old folks". I guess if you look back in time, sometimes the old-folks on the farm lost their shirts and had to lose the farm to the bank. Disease is just like having too many bad-crop years in days gone by on the farm. It drains you physically, emotionally, and financially! Like everything else, money is one driving force of the impact of this disease although I do suspect that it is not just this disease. In every care situation, everyone says that we are so sorry about your wife's condition…now how do you intend to pay for this service. Therefore, money is a driving force in dealing with every aspect of this disease from beginning to end. Just the waiting grace periods for Medicare and Social Security to kick-in can drain your bank account. Not being able to afford a supplemental insurance plan will again drain your bank account. Not having the correct living conditions to deal with wheel chairs, (no stairs, wider doors, ramps etc.) can be a significant added expense. Not having "Long Term Health care insurance" relegates family and friends to be care-givers. Otherwise, your loved one has a pre-existing condition, making it hard just to receive health insurance. If you have financially planned for a terminal illness…you're a step-up. Otherwise, get ready to be stressed about where your next house payment is going to come from!! Let me tell you…the disease will provide all the stress you can handle…period!

Kenni always took care of the bills…again I mowed lawns. Her forte is "head of the family". I really liked this about her. I made an excellent support person. Great, what a team and in fact we are. Through our life Kenni convinced me to continually move houses building our equity. She convinced me to adopt a beautiful daughter, have dogs and that means many and roving in the house, arrange for our younger son to move to New Zealand, arrange for our daughter to attend art school, arrange for our older son to learn a trade, get a horse for our daughter, take long trips to other continents. Then guess what, she still had a teaching career and made money as well! I always said there is nothing better than a strong, smart, good looking woman who makes money! What a love affair!

As you can see, there was a role reversal taking place un-beknownst to me. Whether we wanted to or not, our roles in the family were making huge shifts, shifts that both of us are neither prepared for nor comfortable with. I might also add that roles were beginning to change with our children as well, more on that later. At this time fear sets in! Kenni manifests this fear by crying all the time. Mike's fear manifests itself in crying, in private of course, and a growing anger at everyone and everything. Yelling became the norm. This is my way of dealing with the fear of the unknown and a total feeling of helplessness, and lack of being able to fix this.

Nothing works,
The symptoms march on,
Leaving a path of broken hearts in its path
How do you move on?

Well it appears as though the financial security planning was complete and now we wait and see how well we did. My guess is that the best made plans are always not spot-on! In the midst of the disease, planning becomes difficult. You are forced to be in a constant reactive mode. You are just waiting for the next symptom to appear. We of course knew that we would not live forever, but considering the "good genes" in both families, we anticipated that we would live to a ripe old age. I would submit that if we had done "any" senior/retirement planning, much of the frustration and fear we encountered would have not happened.

Kenni used to always say "you play the cards you're dealt". Guess what, one never really knows what that means. I think it's one way to respond to seeing other people struggle with a disease, sickness, and turmoil. But never the less, at the time it conveys strength about dealing with an unknown. As long as you're healthy, it's just words about something that has not happened. Kenni's last passion was working for the Larch Mountain Prison system teaching GED to inmates. She loved this job, since you did not have to deal with parents. If the "kids" screwed up, they went back to their cells. Most of the time, they really wanted to learn since their release required a GED. In any event, Kenni's forte…teaching people to weather life… were her second passion. It was always rewarding since most came back afterwards and said: "Mrs. Spencer I am so glad to have had you as a teacher and I am glad you were the ultimate Gestapo lady insuring that we really learned, not just pretending too".

In the early stages of ALS, you would notice small changes beginning to take place. There was always hope that at some point the changes would stop or slow down. The medical community would say that about 10% of ALS victims can live longer than 10 years. Hearing that at this stage seemed very comforting. Thinking further about it and how fast 10 years goes, places you back on the worry track.

It became very clear in June of 2009 that this career era was to end for Kenni. The coup-de-grace was when she had to ask one of the inmates to open the locked cabinets in the teaching room. You never give keys to inmates!! The other was that her speech was beginning to slur and communication was becoming a challenge. Finally, just driving there was challenging...how about turning the key on for the car to get there and home? My dad made a gadget for the key making it easier to turn the car on and off. Since we did have a diagnosis, our process was to deal with what came along...not necessarily plan. So Kenni elected to take her third teaching retirement and say good bye. I don't think anyone of us in the family really knew how hard this was for her. After 40+ years of teaching she and I realized that we had to hunker in and spend time fighting this evil disease together. A really scary thought!

Kenni's second retirement from Battleground High School ended in providing a true retirement reward...a real professional quilting machine. She established a home quilting business, Dog Star Farm and was making and selling quilts. The new house we moved to in Washougal, WA was termed our "retirement home". It had a separate building we called the quilt house...small but perfect for her quilting business. I could always tell where Kenni was by seeing the light on in the quilt house. More and more the quilt house was dark. As time went on in 2009 the light never went back on.

I really wanted to see the light back on and quilts being made. I made a plea to the family for someone to step up and have Kenni teach them the quilting machine's nuances. No one showed any interest. So I thought why not me. One late fall day in 2009, we slowly made our way down the curved path to the quilt house. Kenni was to teach me the whole quilting process. Actually, it was quite relaxing and I began to understand why she enjoyed quilting so much. I made it as far as changing the bobbin on the small sewing machine, a necessary tool…and really screwed this apparatus up. The teaching process stopped in its tracks. Kenni said "well, let's go back up to the house, we will come back later". You see she could not "hands-on" show me how to change the bobbin and now the small sewing machine needed to be taken to repair. She could not do that either.

I heard her say…"let's sell the quilting machine"! We never went back down to the quilt house. The machine is up for sale. There were many crying moments for Kenni that I did not see. Her dream of expanding her quilt house for training sessions and sharing her very talented craft with friends, family, and strangers is never to be realized.

A brain in a chair can't quilt,
Oh see the quilting process,
Just can't make it happen,
Cry and cry, and cry more.

As time does march on, each person's life in the family was changing. For me being an "every day Joe" husband was moving to paying bills, running errands, mowing, cleaning, cooking, dog feeding, and providing physical care to Kenni, and a bunch of other stuff. Remember, I worked and mowed lawns. All this other stuff, actually the most important for family structure to work, was overwhelming for me. That's when family members began to change and step up. Older son Morgan, always good with numbers, said he would managing the family finances…wow what a relief. I could not manage money in a cookie jar. He also stepped up and quit his job to stay home with Kenni while I was at work during the day. This is outstanding, allowing me to do my passion…make deals but not lots of money. Plus there is nothing better than work to take your mind off tuff-stuff…it only helps a little! One day I did hear Morgan's comment; "I sure would like to get back on the road again".

Our youngest son Gavin and family were 12,000 miles away and so calling every night became the norm. His feelings of helplessness, separated by distance, caused much anxiety personally and with his family. I am sure that the reassuring comments from far away were comforting to Kenni.

Daughter Hilary decided to move back home to spend important time with Kenni and I'd hope help me with the female part of care giving...but really that part does not affect me in the least. But Hilary does not have to know. Hilary's parking lot visits have stopped and she now comes out to the house on a regular basis...it's quite a distance travel for her. What is really nice is to see her tenderness with Kenni's care. Us male types are so abrasive...just think how men towel themselves after a shower...almost rub the hair off. I find it difficult to provide soft tender care mostly since I am not on the receiving end...I could not feel it. I really know this since I see Kenni's facial expressions when I am applying care...wrinkling of the nose and small whimpers, but never a real complaint. I admired this about her strength in dealing with the disease. Kenni would ask for help in getting comfortable, but never complained about having the disease. One thing astonishing about a terminal illness is that the sun continues to rise and set, dogs bark, newspapers get delivered, but your whole life is turned upside down. You feel disoriented and confused. You feel jealous about healthy people walking around laughing and enjoying life...and we are not!

We have truly been dropped into a world of insecurity and change.

ALS affects about 30,000 people each year. Approximately 5% are unlucky enough to obtain this from a hereditary gene. The other 95% is just a random chance. Think of it, like two people who smoked for 50 years…one gets lung cancer the other does not…pure randomness. Does God have something to do with this? Therefore, you could say that it is a rare disease. I really never even knew what ALS was, although I did know what Lou Gehrig's disease was. Well, they are the same. It really is a very "cheap disease" in retrospect to other diseases! Although I think this is up for discussion. The reason is that there is no real effective treatment. There is only one drug approved by the FDA in the mid 1980's and that is it. The American medical community for years has been focused upon providing comfort care in only living with the disease. Taking the FDA approved drug is only touted to provide 3-6 months of life extension at best. The essence of ALS is that the brain releases a chemical called glutamate that facilitates motor neuron stimulation thereby moving muscles. Our brains do this without thinking. ALS is when the brain constantly pumps glutamate out to the motor neurons…the motor neurons are then constantly stimulated. This constant stimulation causes them to overwork themselves. They eventually die from over exertion and once dead the muscle will not move. If the muscle does not move, it atrophy's and starts to shorten thereby crippling the area. Imagine the tongue, which is a muscle, atrophying due to a dead motor neuron. You cannot move it around to eat, can't lick your lips, stick your tongue out at someone, and you can't use it for speech. The mouth then contorts throwing the bite off effecting food chewing. The chin structure shrinks contorting the face. Now apply this concept to all parts of the body!! I am sure you have the visualization now. But always remember, in most cases, the brain is a functioning entity. You can think, imagine, feel, love, dream, hope but you can't move. That's the ALS disease in a nut-shell! Think of being wrapped in cellophane from head to toe… with only holes to breathe and hear, horrible!

The medical community has geared up to only treat symptoms to be able to live with the disease. They have drugs to help with saliva reduction, depression, constipation, infections, and muscle spasms. They have equipment to help deal with cough management, various splints for limbs to prevent constrictions, electric chairs, voice computers for speech, and much more. Most of the drugs create a plethora of side-effects that require attention as well. None of these processes offers any HOPE…just comfort in helping to live with the disease. This is one of the few diseases that if you have it…do what "they" say, go home and get your things in order for certain death. For Kenni and family, this created incredible anxiety and depression…crying became the norm along with incredible mood swings. We never did talk about her fear, but I must believe that it was prevalent. If the medical community could create some sort of HOPE, then living with the disease would be much more tolerable. When you are depressed, hope seems almost unknowable, a total illusion. You tend to go through the motions. Your energy ebbs and your spirits are heavy. At any given time, false hopes are created with alternative treatments…acupuncture, vitamins, lithium, herbs, clinical trials and the like. It's amazing how at the on-set they do give you some level of hope.

But as time progresses, you continue to see the progression and you end up saying…"well that's not working"…depression goes deeper.

Kenni's ALS progression started in her right hand in September of 2008. By May of 2010 it had moved to her left hand, left arm, tongue, feet, neck and legs. There is literally no movement in her hands and arms. She has lost her balance along with her ability to walk. Falling became an everyday occurrence. Our new house rule, "It's not ok to fall". With every fall serious injury always occurred. Her Achilles tendons have shrunk so much that she can't walk on her heels. Her speech is gone and eating has been relegated to soups and pureed/soft foods. She really can't chew things. Swallowing anything including thin liquids like water is a challenge (by the way, they have water thickeners available). With constant choking, you have to be concerned about bacterial pneumonia. Remember muscles move the tongue and throat. As you can see, she requires full care to live each day. Someone needs to help her shower, dress, take liquids, movement from place to place, snot management, saliva management…on and on. I am sure that I have forgotten something.

Ever experienced really needing someone,
Ever waited for the spoon to reach your mouth,
Can't do anything until someone helps,
Not a way to live then you cry

Since ALS with Kenni I have noticed some very important things that cause me to stop and think. As a family our dreams literally have stopped. I have no sleep dreams about Kenni. She has disappeared from my dreams. Why is that? Does that mean that she is in theory dead? Our passions dwindled to one thing…live with ALS as a family. The things that were once important to Kenni and I are no longer important. I don't know if that is something good or not. We used to be very passionate about our surroundings, our life style and home. Entertaining was a real passion being able to share this with family and friends. It is just not important anymore. We don't even talk about it, even if we could. Our passion of communicating with each other through verse and touch has totally changed. I think for me this has been the most difficult. The house remains quite except the TV. Communicating is spelling a few letters of a word for understanding…and it is basic…like "nose"…I know what that means. As the disease has progressed now she just wrinkles her nose…and I know she wants her nose wiped. Kenni can't ask how my day went and did I pick up milk on the way home. She can't say that she loves me and have me understand it. Today she would spell out the word "love". Sure I know, but losing the communication impulse is a huge horrible loss for our relationship on both sides. This is without a doubt the worst part of the disease. It's not only dire on the receiving end, but can you really imagine the frustration on the giving end?

What used to be important is no more,
Life's critical importance, only comfort,
One blink yes two blinks no,
Immense fear of what's next.

On a late September 2010 day, Kenni said that she did not feel right and wanted to go to the hospital. Because of her lack of nutrition and water she was very near death…and I did not even realize it. Her weight was below 100 lbs. I knew she was losing weight, but seeing her every day you lose the relative comparison. She needed a feeding tube and had actually made the decision to have one. This is truly a move of compassion on her part. You probably are asking why? The simple answer is that it was tearing at her heart to watch each family member struggle with feeding her, knowing that she was going to die because of lack of water and food. Kenni made the ultimate choice for her family…and guess what; the feed tube did its job for each family member. The pain of it is the "giving up" of another freedom to the disease.

Kenni's days are relegated to the sofa watching TV with the controller in hand…and she can still manage to change a channel or two. It is truly a "Brain in a Chair". What are you going to do…wait for tomorrow and do the same thing? What else? How do you provide independence for someone in this state? Even Providence Hospital, having one of the best ALS clinics in the US struggles with this management issue. They all have opinions based upon scientific data and experience. And guess what, they go home to healthy families, to my knowledge. This is a job for most and a passion for few. Each family's condition and surroundings are different. Some people with ALS take up and move to a single floor dwelling in the city, thereby being able to get out in to the community. Not really, but the concept is good. What really happens is that there needs to be someone there willing to provide the necessary "movement" and care 100% of the time. That's it very simply. Most who provide this movement and care are family members and a few are friends and lastly strangers in a facility if necessary. The person providing the movement care must be totally committed and have their priorities in the correct place. I have struggled with this…due to my intense anger and sadness. But no time to deal with your personal fears, concerns, and desires…right?

They only get in the way of giving real care. I have truly experienced this first hand. To the person with ALS, like Kenni, movement and the reward of movement is "comfort". Comfort becomes a very important and immediate need.

Nothing else matters at the moment. Change the pillow, wipe my nose, turn my hand over, pull my arms, scratch my forehead, and rub my eyes…on and on. Think of your nose running…you immediately grab for a tissue and take care of it. All done and never give it a second thought. For Kenni, if no one provides the necessary movement action, her nose keeps running down her face into her mouth. It becomes an overwhelming annoyance like water dripping on your forehead. Then there is discomfort. Constant discomfort will eventually cause the disease to cast its grip harder and harder and you start to say…"I think you're worse today than you were yesterday". In fact, you are correct. To help another is to forget for a few moments your own needs. You can gain some comfort in knowing that you are not the only one caring for someone suffering. This care giving notion provides a bond and kinship in ways that only those who have followed in the same shoes can appreciate. He or she has been there. There is also a bond created with the care-giver and patient. Even though there is deep love, care-giving truly transcends this by bringing life-giving hope to another human being as they weather the disease…they are not alone.

For me the caregiver, this ALS event has made me a very angry person...why? A whole bunch of emotions: Why Kenni? Why our family? What did she do or I do to deserve this? Whose fault is it anyway? Why has God allowed this? Things happen for a reason? Are you kidding me! I can see no good or learning coming from this disease. Both Kenni and I are not going to become better people because of this experience. Do you really think that we will? Maybe there is a reason in which we just don't know nor will understand in this life time? Who can I blame? I need to blame someone or something! I need to understand why this has happened to our family...because ALS victims are everyone surrounding Kenni...our family, our friends, and even strangers. My anger is directed towards myself, Kenni, the medical community, insurance companies, the Government and God. Now you can tell me I am crazy and I need to have some psychological help or support and you may be right. Do you know of a good therapist? But who is right...first walk in my shoes then let me know what you feel and think. It appears as though everyone has an opinion on how to act and behave when dealing with a disease. Many a news paper columnist has written about many people dealing with terminal illnesses and the good that has come from it!! Emotional journalism regarding terminal illness is rampant in every news paper every day. If it is not a warm feel-good story about an important person with terminal disease and cause, then it's just another OBIT. Everyone professionally and as a layman, seems to know what to tell a person with ALS and the family...here is what you need to do... now go do it!

Tell me how to act,
Immediate and growing anger,
Self pity look inward,
How would they behave with the same hand dealt,
Hugging and understanding.

As this disease cripples Kenni, at the same time it cripples the family dynamics. At the pinnacle of our family are ALS and Kenni. Everything revolves around the disease. Yet, sons, daughters, grand children, parents, and friends have their own lives to live. Who is interested in this? Who wants to hear constantly about ALS in the Spencer family? Who cares! Why don't we talk about our children's dreams and accomplishments? Why don't we get back to having small talk about and with our friends? Why has it become so hard to ask your friends, what's been happening in your lives? How is your son or daughter doing? Say, Dave, how is business? These questions and discussions literally stop for the most part. ALS has made our family only one dimensional now. The daily living dynamic has shrunk to our selfishness. Maybe this is right? I don't know. Maybe this is what "fighting a disease" is all about. Maybe this is an urging by others to "talk about it" to feel comfortable.

ALS has driven our family to operate under the regime of "routine". Once you move out of the daily routine, there is fear and discomfort. Think about it; get Kenni out of the house into the community, what an event. There is the fear of something going wrong, falling, embarrassment, explanation. It is so much easier to stay at home, eat, watch TV, read...no problems. You ever watch people look at a "Brain in a Chair"? There is total over reaction to help, starring, impatience, pity, and a reluctance to engage. I see it every time we are out. How do you communicate with someone who can't talk? The truth...you talk, share love, hug, rub the arm, read a book to them...that's probably the best thing. This does not happen most of the time, because we are all wrapped up in our personal agendas, "the me" syndrome. That's the way it is! I could be wrong here, but spending time with a "Brain in a Chair" clearly takes people out of their comfort zone. And you know what; one really can't blame them for not spending time with a person with ALS. It is a very uncomfortable sobering experience.

Be around ALS,
Really uncomfortable,
What do you say, what do you do,
Silence silence silence,
Can't wait to go home.

Therefore, providing care and living a normal life can't happen. They are incongruent. Life for the Spencer family is not normal now nor will it ever be. A family member recently said…"I wish things could be like they used to"! We certainly would like this, but in reality, life keeps throwing changes. It's how you deal with these changes that can enrich your family life. Is that the right thing to say? I think that this is the right thing to say. But this becomes a very hard task for me. Change has always been hard. The change caused by ALS has crippled my spirit. I will never be the same nor will any other family member. But we do have each other! But what does that mean? We are fearful of the future and life without Kenni, the family rock. The only thing left is memories, and lately they are not nice memories. I guess we need to be thankful having known the victim of ALS throughout their whole life and memories of the good times and days gone by. The ALS disease is only one portion of the life cycle.

Remember when we did,
Remember when we laughed,
Remember when we loved,
The best! The best!

This last phase is probably the most important.
Family and friends is the only hook that ALS
victims have to latch onto. As the disease
progresses, the real friends tend to weed themselves
out. Even family members begin to argue more
amongst themselves. All family members have a
different experience than me, and sometimes we
stumble over one another, hurt one another, and
feel hurt ourselves. Again it is really all about
comfort zones. We tend to gravitate towards things
that we feel comfortable with. No one feels
comfortable around someone who is sick. It tugs at
your heart strings. What do you say to make them
feel better? What do you do to make them feel
better? How do you just pass the time? Can you
help? "Whoops… got to go"! That's normal.
In the beginning of the disease friends were inviting
us to entertainment venues; family events were
spontaneous, girl's day out, etc. As time goes on
these become less and less. The progressive states of
the disease clearly cause this. What a shame. Pretty
soon you are whittled down to just a few friends
and family and very few sharing moments. These
people are the true troopers. Real friends and
family! You know who you are.
I think that there is a need to honor the sanctity of
our own space and the need for others to be
present…for love, company, for understanding and
support!

These real family and friends do stand-out as real and caring. Think of this…just sit quietly with Kenni or maybe read a book to her. Not complicated, but very hard to do. What a revelation! How meaningful on both sides. I know because I have seen it work. How about painting her nails or giving hand and arm rubs.

You then take notice about everyone's comments and facial expressions. Are these true and real? When they say they are sorry you have this terrible disease…are they really? I would offer to you that this is just the "politically correct" thing to say. It's a win-win feel good position. They have done their part and can now go home to their healthy families. Am I really being fair here…who knows? I would propose to you that a very "jealous" attitude has crept into my psyche. It is the old notion that the first wealth is health…they're in good health and we aren't.

Love and care,
Be true to yourself,
Help those that can't help themselves,
Spend time, meaningful time,
There always is an end!

These are hard words to hear because our impulse is to withdraw from other people. They are carrying on their ordinary lives when our world has fallen apart. How can they understand? Besides, our sadness will make them uncomfortable. I suppose we need to resume our place in the human family!

The final chapter of the disease is oriented towards end of life care and that's it. What does that really mean? Each ALS victim is encouraged to fill out a "POLST" form defining your end of life care preferences. This is a legal binding document signed by your doctor. If you go into cardiac arrest…what methods of life care do you want…ventilator, feeding tube, antibiotics, etc.? This is very tough stuff to put down on paper. It defines the reality of your situation. But, we did it! Since Kenni already had a feeding tube, she elected to continue nourishment and antibiotics if there were infections. That was it! My desire was totally different. I of course wanted every measure to keep her here on the planet…guess what? This is not my body and my life. It leaves the family members with such a feeling of hopelessness and total lack of control. Panic and anger really set in since the reality of the situation has been clarified. For Kenni, it created a calming, since it was one very small step in maintaining control over this evil disease.

The disease takes away,
The disease gives nothing back,
Your decisions give back control.
I can now rest.

Our attempts to "be brave" and "keep a stiff upper lip", is a false pretense.

Since she had elected to not have a ventilator, breathing was more and more of an issue. It was one Sunday afternoon, friends had left and Kenni said that she wanted to go to the Hospital. She could not breathe. I contacted her doctor and she referred to the "POLST" form and said…"Mr. Spencer, there is nothing that we can do, other than to move your wife into the Hospice system". You know, I have heard of this from friends and TV advertisements. The overwhelming response was that they are wonderful, and the TV ads showed smiling people. So, Hospice it was and they responded quickly…why is that? Is it a competitive business? I don't know. In any event, getting Kenni signed up tugged at my heart strings. They ask you questions, "Does she have a PEG (feed tube)"? Of course, the response was…"yes". Their response was that they could not accept her, since there mission was "end of life care" and the feeding tube was considered extending life. I was shocked and could not believe what I was hearing. I got very upset and said that even with the feeding tube, Kenni was going to die. They indicated that they would have to have a meeting with the area supervisor for a decision. At this point I am so-o-o-o frustrated with the bureaucracy of the disease. Why does this have to happen? After phone calls to doctors and health care specialists, they elected to "enroll" Kenni into Hospice. Once you elect to move into Hospice, you must sign-out of Hospital/Clinic. You can't have both! I don't know why, but I bet it has something to do about the entities getting paid…"green backs". In doing this you really feel like you're leaving home. All that you have known and anticipated is gone. You are entering a new home...an un-easy feeling for everyone involved. Don't get me wrong, Hospice has good components of care…in particular, the nurses. They are qualified and loving people. They can be an excellent resource to tap into. They can provide the needed guidance and professional support as the disease continues its final grip. They also have a team of volunteers, who contact you on a regular basis for support. However, I found that this level of support was not helpful for us. Kenni needed to have her mouth suctioned out every 15 minutes and they were not qualified or allowed to do this type of task. Therefore, the volunteer group could not be alone with her and help take the burden off of us for a short time… but, they can bathe her…I don't get that.

After all our attempts to make sense out of this hospice dying thing, we are left with a huge hole in the fabric of our lives. I feel like I am being in perpetual danger of falling into the astonishing abyss of Kenni's death. Not wanting to let go at first is one of the compromises. I am forced to make decisions with helping prepare her end of life care. Perhaps I have become Kenni's guardian angel!

It was a rainy day as the Hospice nurse was checking kenni. She turned to me and asked if I had made any funeral arrangements.

For me, doing that was admitting defeat to the disease. It was totally a reality check that my "love" was going to die. This was a constant approach-avoidance through-out her disease progression. You know that by making funeral arrangements, this was the last step…absolutely no hope. I would submit that another difficult aspect of this disease to deal with…there is no hope. Why is the Medical community continually telling you that there is always hope? Where was it hiding?? Please explain to us just what this "hope" is.

When you enter into Hospice, they provide a book explaining all the services and everything you want to know but are afraid to ask. In particular, one pamphlet, charts the symptoms of death, separated into months, weeks, days, and hours. Why have this available? I found that this really tugged at my heart strings and I certainly was not going to share this with Kenni. None of the family wanted to know how much longer that our loved one was going to be here on the planet. All I could see this creating is more fear of the future. Regardless, we tried to capture each day and hour spending the best quality of time with Kenni that we could. Some days Kenni and I seem to be managing well, confident that we can face the future. There are other times that we both feel abandoned and left in a dark room alone…the times are dark now.

One month to go difficulting breathing,
One day to go disconnecting from the world,
One hour to go feet and hands blue,
One minute to go shallow breadths,
One last breadth…gone

Has this writing journey helped me, I am not sure, but maybe some. Will I survive this journey? I don't know for sure. I am extremely fearful of "what's next". My heart is very sick and my psyche is damaged. Please don't tell me that with time you will get better. Please don't share with me that there is a grief process that family and friends will go through. I guess the only thing I can offer is that I have gained a new compassion for people who are sick and stuck with life changing events beyond their control. God help me and them and I hope that I stay in step.

In sharing this, I hope that it has opened up your eyes to dealing with terminal illness from a regular everyday family. Thanks!

Kenni flew away from this world on May 30, 2011 from ALS.

Dearest Kenni,
Let it not be death but completeness,
Let love melt into memory and pain into songs,
Let the flight through the sky end in the folding of your wings over your nest,
Let the last touch of your hands be gentle like the flower of the night,
Stand still, O beautiful end for a moment, and say your last words in silence,
I bow to you Kenni and hold up my lamp to light you on your way.
TaGore

Mike Spencer
ALS in Partnership.

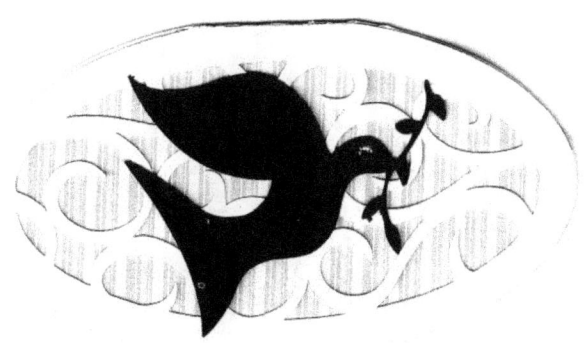